IF I CAN DO IT YOU CAN TOO

WEIGHT LOSS MOTIVATION & TIPS

RITU DUBEY

Contents

Foreword

This is my journey and I am really proud of everything including my failures. I failed and I learnt from it and failure is a part of every journey. I want to dedicate this book completely to my husband as he was the only person who never body shamed me or made me feel depressed. He supported me throughout this journey and also allowed me to dream of this picture today.

If you are a man and you are reading this book then understand the woman whoever she is be it your wife, sister, mother or for that matter anyone just let her know that you are with her. It's not about weight loss, rather support her in all her dreams and goals. I know today that everything is possible just because of my husband who supported me in my weird plans, allowed me to workout while he took care of our child, paid for all those expensive gym equipment and even helped me pursue my nutrition course. I am self-sufficient today and financially independent but if it wasn't for him I wouldn't have been here and writing this book.

I just want you all to know that like our fingerprints we have different bodies too and instead of comparing yourself to others try to work on your own self and look for ways how you can feel better than yesterday. This book is a guide on how you can change your mindset and can see fitness as a lifetime goal.

You are not born to fit a dress size, goals should be real and try to work on your inner peace which is way too important. Happy reading!!

CHAPTER ONE

Trying Hard To Be Perfect

When it comes to beauty standards in women we all picture a woman with perfect curves, toned legs, firm breast, smaller waist, flawless skin and knee long hair. Since our childhood, whenever we have looked at women with those looks and admired them, I believe that we all girls somewhere in our heart want to look exactly like that. It's not our mistake, actually this is the societal norms in which we have grown up and we all want to be accepted as being beautiful.

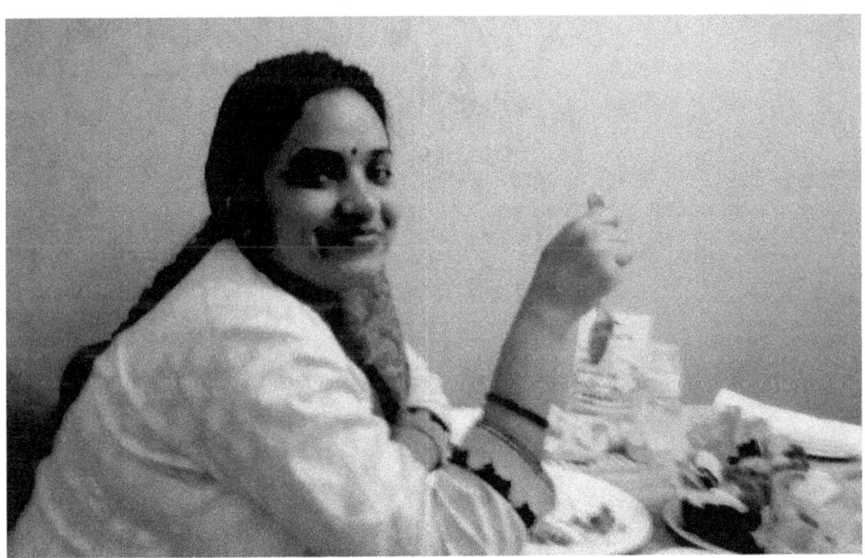

This Is Me - Heavy But Still Happy

So here I am breaking the norms and telling you my story how I was being skinny fat since my childhood & then gained oodles of pregnancy weight, became obese post pregnancy, looked in the eyes with sympathy by almost everyone including my parents, suffered major health issues, did all sort of diets available online or through guidance but atlast accepting that this is my body with which I was born and have to ultimately die with and there came this drastic change. You know what? I fell in love with me the way I never loved anyone else and the story changed.

This book is for each one of you whether you are a school going teenager or a college going girl, whether you are married or have grandkids to play with. This book will help you to realise how important it is to understand and love your own body as we all are flawed humans and just because you are a few kgs heavier doesn't mean you have to abandon or hate yourself.

Before we begin with my journey let me tell you we all are different and so are our bodies so stop wishing or comparing yourself to anyone out there. Just read this book not at one time but keep it handy and read it until and unless you really understand the message behind it.

CHAPTER TWO

Have We Changed?

I have seen my mother and my aunts having those beautiful bodies which we really crave for these days. Back then they ate everything including oil, ghee and sugar but their waist line was so small and they had such an appealing body irrespective of how many kids they have reproduced. My grandmother looked super hot and even in her 70s her skin glowed like a 30 year old girl without any wrinkles or ageing signs and she never ever visited any salon for her hair and skin treatment. Forget about the dermatologist, she only went to the hospital when she was badly sick during the last days of her life, she even delivered all her kids at home. I have been thinking about this a lot and now it makes some sense to me about the food, nutrition and lifestyle which impacted a lot in their times and of course the pollution too.

If you just go 20 years back and try to look at eating habits you could actually see everything has changed a lot and for that matter the weight loss industry grew big and big and our local farmers are now dying because no one is willing to pay them the cost of their products. I am not here to question or judge who is right and who is wrong, I am just trying to point out where we actually went wrong and I realised all of this after going through all on my own. In the name of modernisation we have completely given up on our food habits, eating local food and moreover we need a trained person (dietitian/nutritionist) to guide us how much and what to eat.

Previously food was considered as a goddess and that is why we never tried to discard any food and left over was also used by the families and we followed those rituals religiously as our soul was connected to it but as we started getting modern not only dining tables were introduced but also different sorts of diets came into play. Now we don't look at food as any god/goddess but we look at it with calories, proteins and carbohydrates. More we started experimenting with our eating habits, the more problems increased and of course the number of diseases as well. We don't eat sugar because it has blank calories, we don't eat rice because it has bad carbohydrates/starch, we don't include ghee in our diet because it contains fat that will turn us into an obese. We have gathered so much knowledge through the internet that we simply deny all the knowledge which was given to us or passed on to us by our forefathers or prior generations. This is not just weight loss, it's about our complete ignorance and lack of knowledge that we are into so much trouble.

We don't eat right and then we face hair fall issues and to fix that we and go see one doctor. Then we have skin breakouts and we visit another one. We also get different sort of hormonal imbalance which is directly connected to our diet and so we hit the clinic of one more doctor and hence the list goes on. I am a small town girl and I never heard of gym, aerobics, zumba in my childhood days as my daughter is seeing me now doing everyday may be I will also set an example for her.

I am not saying gym is bad but still think how people managed to look good in those days and had a much better life at least in terms of mental peace. I can bet my mother never went to any fitness centre but she did all household chores on her own and she can still do whatever she feels like. Her hair is waist long and doesn't talk about volume because even I dont have half of what she has and yes her secret is that she applies coconut oil and shampoos once a week and for that she gets her hair colored at home with the help of our househelp. I have got her genes but all my habits are different and yes I have been through all like hair fall, acne, PCOS, thyroid and what else. I have been to many doctors, dermatologists, trichologists, cosmetologists and spent a huge amount of money but now I am back to basics. I am doing exactly what my mother and my grandmother did and yes I could see the change though still there is a long way to go and I know I will be there soon.

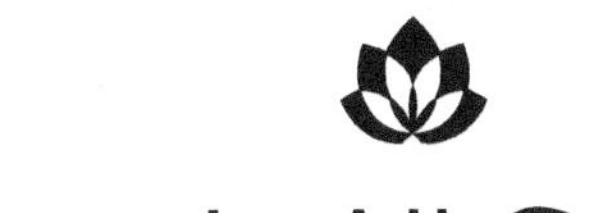

CHAPTER THREE

How It All Started

First thing first, respect and love your body and this line is something we all should use as a mantra day in and day out. If we don't love our own self how can we even expect others to? I have not been a very lean girl throughout my childhood and people kept bullying me everywhere so I always hated myself for looking that way which was by the way skinny fat like a chubby kid. Many complimented me saying that I have an hourglass or mermaid body but somewhere I never accepted myself. I kept blaming myself for looking in such a way that everyone looked at me, I wasn't fat but genetically body type was good enough to take everyone's attention towards it. So throughout my childhood I just looked at my Barbie doll and believed that one day I will achieve a body like this.

Back then in the 90's the Internet was not so popular though I had a dial up connection at home which took forever to connect to the internet and my computer was in my father's room so he always kept an eye on what I was doing so I never got a chance to enhance my knowledge on weight loss and bodybuilding. I was focusing more on my studies because that is what we were supposed to do to keep our parents happy. I remember having breakfast before going to school was mandatory which used to be banana and a glass of milk sometimes other fruits which were available in the season, lunch boxes were used to be like paratha sabji or stuffed parathas and lunch used to be rice (in small quantity), dal with ghee, any vegetable curry and a roti with ghee along with salad and raita ofcourse.

I played a lot of sports during my school time and yes I believe that helped me to build up good stamina. Evenings were mostly milk and biscuits or chapati with ghee and jaggery in it, which is still my favorite and dinner used to be around 7 PM and that too very light. When I was at home I never had any hair fall issues or skin breakouts and was not even obese and starving was never an option because my mother never allowed any such non sense because for her those were my growth years and she was feeding me exactly what I needed the most. I could easily recall that whenever we went to our native's place my grandmother offered us jaggery with water as that was something homemade and in the evening snack she used to give us sattu (grounded black chana) in the water with some black salt and jeera powder in it and that tasted wonders and of course she used to put so much ghee in our food stating this is the purest form of love.

During summers we used to visit our mango farms and we could eat as much as we wanted to and trust me guys I literally survived on mangoes because I really love them and I never felt constipated, bloated or gained weight. It felt so good to be sitting with the entire family and enjoying the family time with mangoes.

Today I can speak about all of this because I have learnt a lot now and don't worry I didn't learn it until I got my own lesson and that too a very hard one. So after my school life got over and I went to college I decided to join a fitness club to transform myself. Initially it felt good as I just used to walk on treadmills or ride a cycle, like I was more into cardio and for me weight training was something not meant for girls so I never took the pain to even look into the weighing section. I started working out in 2009 and yes I felt good as doing something is always better than nothing. But I never had the motivation to go to the gym regularly, I used to go like once or twice a week and I used to create excuses like I have to study a lot, I can't afford any time to waste, I am in good shape I don't need to exercise daily, I will do it regularly from next week which never came.

It was not only me who was thinking that weights are for male. I believe almost everyone felt the same way and so mostly all women/females were into cardio. After wasting a complete year membership I decided to hire a personal trainer and so I did. He taught me how to use weights and how to target different muscles in our body. For the first time in my life I was getting to know that my leg is not just leg it has glutes, hamstrings, calves into it and so I really felt good though initially weight training gives you trouble like you will get sore, you won't be able to move and you will feel like giving up as it looks like complete torture.

Nowadays you can get motivation from social media itself as everyone is doing it so why can't I but at that time there was no concept of comparing your life on social media, I believe there was this orkut and nothing else. Anyways, I was doing well with my trainer and he really helped me a lot and he was the first one who introduced me to the word "DIET". One day during the training sessions I told him I can't see much changes in my body to which he asked me to tell him about my diet, for the first few seconds I just looked at him and then I said okay so you are asking me about my eating habits and food to which he said yes. I told him my entire day's eating plan to which he said you are taking too many carbohydrates and that is why you can't see any results. You need to add more protein to your diet, skip your dinner and then you can see the change.

I am a pure vegetarian girl from a brahmin family and I knew that the best protein sources were meat and eggs so I asked how I can get enough protein? He said you can easily get it through protein powder which I can get for you. So now I was introduced to the first supplement in my life which was growing with the weight loss industry. I never had any idea or money so I went to my dad and told him the same. He said a big NO and told me to focus more on studies than the gym. I thought he was right because I was not going to make a career out of it. I never had any idea that one day the fitness industry would be on sky 9 or else I would have also stuck with the fitness industry only. But yes after my trainer told me about skipping my dinner so I thought of trying it. Initially I had to face a lot of problems because my body looked for dinner and I just used to have a glass of milk or maybe lemon water thinking this would help me in a long way but that was the worst thing I did to myself.

CHAPTER FOUR

How We Grow Up Ignoring Fitness

Now I believe we should always do something which we can do forever for the rest of our life but at that point of time to me my trainer was the knowledge box and to me whatever he said was absolutely right and something I must adhere to without questions. Skipping dinners for a month actually helped me with weight loss but apart from taking those numbers down it also gave me good dark circles around my eyes and my stamina also reduced, I felt lethargic throughout the day, my concentration reduced a lot and I started cravings biscuits and indian sweets and I also never had any energy to work out.

My parents got concerned as for them it was something very alarming and they took me to a doctor for a thorough check up. Doctor told them where I was going wrong and gave me some multivitamin tablets. My father got angry and asked me to discontinue from the fitness club, I really had no choice left so I had to do what he said. I stayed home and focused more on my studies. Going out with friends became regular and so binging on junk foods also. It's not something I wanted to indulge in but at times you can't say no to your friends because you can't explain the reason and we never had any healthy alternatives to consider back then. We preferred Indian snacks more than anything else and I believe the obesity rate in India was pretty less back then.

During our teenage years our metabolism is pretty high and digestion really works very well. As we start growing up we move less and eat more. That is the major reason we grow big on our waist line. The bottom line is our body is meant to move so just don't spend your entire day sitting at your workplace trying to move in every half an hour to an hour at least for a minute.

Have you ever noticed that the rickshaw pullers or our house helps gaining fat or their kids becoming obese. It's not because they don't eat much, it's because they live their life with the basic principles. They wake up early in the morning, do all their household chores and then come to your place do everything at your place and eat whatever you give them and then again they go back to their place and eat early dinner and then they sleep early so that they wake up early the next morning. Same goes with the rickshaw or cart pullers. They lift their body weights along with others and ride the cycle. They want to do maximum rounds so that they can go back home with good money for their dinner. They don't have a social media account to compare their lives with others, they don't have friends to socialise with or go to bar with, they can't afford lavish dinners or can't make it out to any restaurant, they live on their daily wage and just eat what they get and are hardly found with any sort of emotional or mental health problems.

You know we have a problem. We feel good to show off like eating imported berries instead of indian gooseberry which is a great source of vitamin C, banana is a complete food in itself but as it is cheap so we ignore it and we switch to imported apples or kiwis, we want to prove with our behaviour everywhere that I can afford it because I have got so much money. It looks so classy to have 3 househelps at home and one nanny to look after our own kid and spending your entire day on a couch by just looking at others life on social media and feeling depressed about it.

Social media is a box full of lies everyone post just to show how good they are doing in their life not to share their happiness just to make others feel that their life is so unworthy. You see fitness models doing ad of certain products and people getting so much influenced that they instantly buy it without giving a second thought to it. Do you think anyone would come up to show the dark secrets of their life or how tough life is for them? It's good to be connected with others but not at the stake of your own mental health. Remember never compare your life to others because we all are different from each other and one should never ever compare themselves to anyone else.

I am not against social media, actually it's the reverse. I believe social media is a blessing for those who know how to make proper use of it and a curse for those who get into it and lose themselves just looking at others and how great their life is. This is the best platform to grow and learn at the same time but not by keeping your peace at stake. There is a trend going on these days that people come up with some great transformation pictures and yell about how they lost so much weight and if you want to know how they achieved it then start following them or pay them for personal coaching and people just follow them blindly without even giving a second thought to it.

No one on this earth can help you if you are not willing to help yourself and keep in mind that what might work for one person may not work for others as we all have different bodies and the way you have eaten foods depending on your birth place or your climatic conditions, medical history, genetics, lifestyle, etc. needs to be taken well care of and so if you cannot afford a certified nutritionist or dietitian then you are your best dietitian. I always knew when I was eating wrong, when I didn't workout properly and everything but I chose to ignore because I was looking for certain magic to happen. I always had a belief till I am able to get my dress size in the market I shouldn't be much bothered about my weight or anything else. We have to shun this behavior while we are young. Fitness is a lifetime process and the early you start, the better fit you will be for all your life.

CHAPTER FIVE

Marriage, Pregnancy & Weight Gain

After my graduation I gained a few kgs and decided to go for Zumba certification as that was the best way not just to lose weight but also to make a career out of it. I continued as I was very good at dance so my interest kept me attached to Zumba classes. I couldn't make my career out of it as I got married at an early age. Marriage at an early age was a complete shock in itself as you have to adjust with everyone and you barely know them. My in-laws were of a pretty conservative mindset though my husband wasn't like them and like every other girl gaining weight post marriage I started doing the same. The best part of my body is that it works on LIFO (last in first out), that is, every time I gain weight it comes first on the butts and thigh and last on my face but whenever I lose those extra weight it's my face which loses it first and at last from my thighs and butts.

Within 3 months of my marriage when I was just eating, cooking and having fun I got pregnant which was very accidental but in Indian societies this is termed as the best news. I realised that it's time that I need to forget and give up on my dreams and carry on with this baby as this would be my life now and really it sounds great but it isn't. Giving up your entire life and goals being a housewife and raising kids was something I never had in my mind. But pregnancy brings so much joy in our life. But along with that it also brings tough times to the mother who is carrying her child inside her womb. To me my pregnancy was the toughest as I had morning sickness throughout nine months, for that matter I would say whenever I ate something I just used to throw it out. Initially I felt so sick that I never felt like getting out of my bed but after a month or so I decided to move around as it doesn't help much.

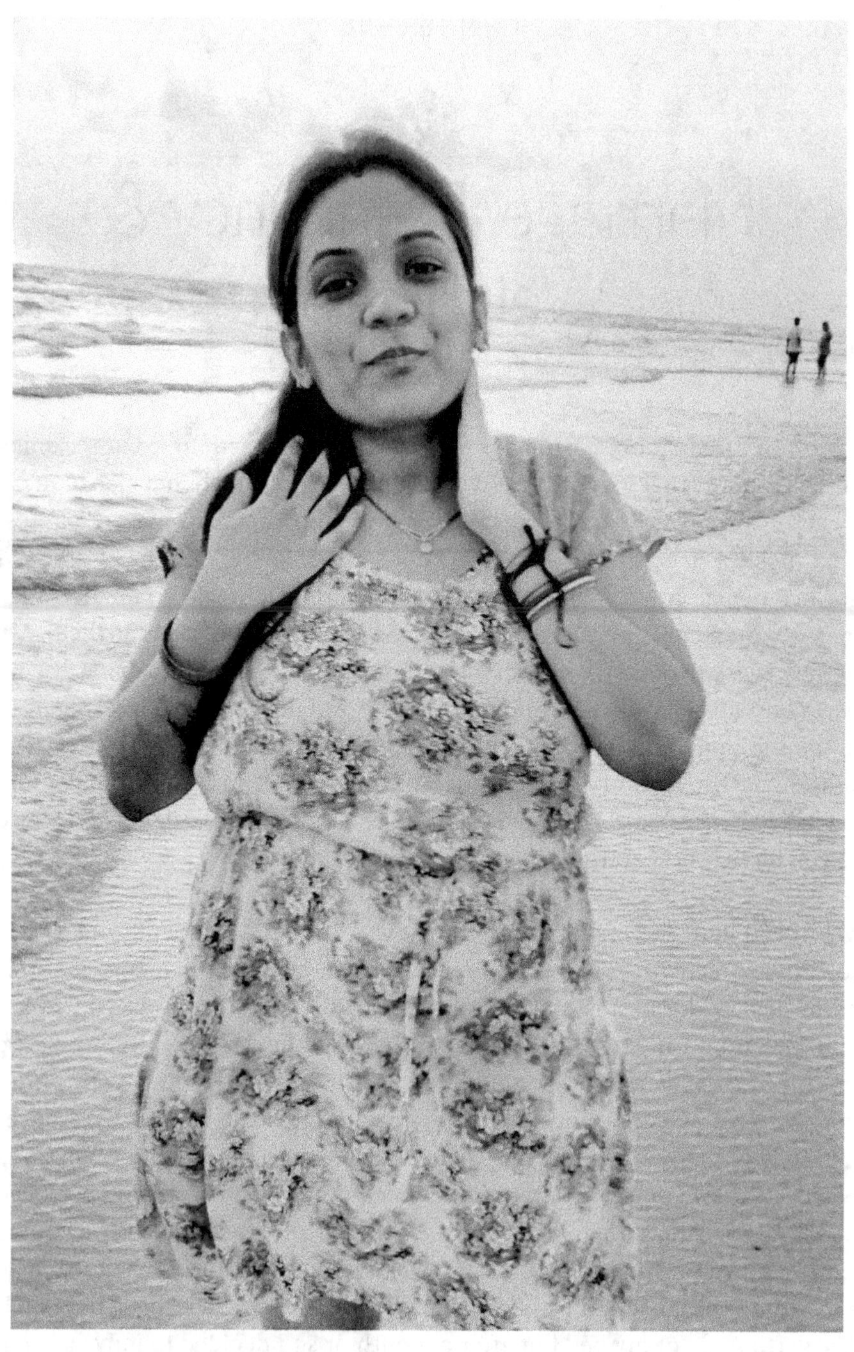

Me Enjoying The Pregnancy

My mother in law started feeding me excess ghee in everything along with dry fruits ladoo as she wanted me to deliver a very healthy baby and she always used to remind me that i should eat for two which is a complete misconception as you just need to eat nutritious food as much as you can digest and according to your appetite. I don't know about the baby but yes I was gaining weight very quickly, I just won't blame ghee and dry fruits ladoo for that matter, I even had to tempt my taste buds. It is said if you feel the urge to eat something then you should not suppress it. So I did exactly what was explained to me and my biggest cravings were Pizza with cold drinks, chocolates and loads of ice creams. I never took any note of my nutritional requirements or calorie intake. I just ate everything I craved for and then threw up most of the time. My gynaecologist was pretty concerned as I was gaining more than enough and I had no control over my food temptations.

I believe in a span of 3 months I was already 15-20 kgs heavier than my normal body weight. Looking at my weight my doctor asked me to involve myself in some sort of physical activity. So I bought a treadmill as going out for a walk was not a good choice for me and I even did some sort of pregnancy yoga. But when you see your belly and body growing together you don't feel much motivation to exercise and the same was happening to me. My junk food intake was increasing day by day and with each passing day my discomfort started to increase. I lost control of my bladder and this made me stay awake at night to urinate every now and then and so I got a chance to indulge into late night snacking as well and as my husband was my partner in crime so it used to be either instant noodles, chips or some cookies.

Doctor kept warning me that this weight gain was pretty alarming and that I was growing up very quickly in the second trimester only and was not much focused on my health and fitness. I could realise something was happening inside me as I had digestion issues and kept throwing up all day and night but I thought it happens during pregnancy and as it was my very first child I really had no idea about all of this. Going to my gynaecologist and getting regular check ups was something that was pretty regular and irrespective of my confusions I never shared or asked her anything because everyone told me that your body will entirely change just go through this phase and enjoy it. I thought I was doing well until one day I realised I started to feel itchy all over my body, I spoke to my mother and she said that's fine it just happens.

But day by day it became worse and I was scratching myself very badly. I could feel the itch everywhere inside my nails, on the soles of my feet, on my back everywhere. I took baths several times a day and even applied different sorts of lotions but nothing helped. So when I had exhausted all my options I spoke to my doctor for the same and she got my LFT (Liver Functioning Test) done and to my surprise yes there was some problem with my liver. She told me as I was in my second trimester and the medications could affect my baby so she told me to take good care of myself and gave certain medicines to suppress the itching. She clearly told me that after delivery I need to get back to my medications so that my liver can be treated well. Her medication did help but it could not help me to get rid of the itching completely.

I am married to a family who believes that cooking should be done by daughter in law only so I had a house help who did the cleaning of the house and utensils only and rest was done by me. I never complained about anything and did all the household chores including washing of the clothes. Whenever my doctor asked me about my delivery I wanted to go with the normal one and that is why I was doing pelvic exercises throughout my pregnancy.

As I was not very close to my MIL being a newlywed I decided to deliver my baby at my parents place so I went back home in 7 month though I had a hard time travelling but yes that was something I wanted for my own comfort. Staying with my mother helped her to feed me what she thought was right for the baby and I looked more like a balloon and used to walk like a duck all the time as my tummy was way too big and my legs also. I never thought I would gain so much weight in my life!

CHAPTER SIX

Baby Coming & Body Shaming

After struggling straight for 8 months I went to see the appointed delivery doctor for the last scan where he informed me that I will be operated on for the due date which was just fifteen days away as there was not much water left for the movement of the baby so he will perform a C-Section to take my child out. One more thing I would like to tell you all that on the day of my last scan I was at 99 kgs and the doctor looked at me as if he had never seen these digits before. He laughed and even said that you can make it 100 by the time of your delivery with a sarcastic tone but who cares. I went home and got really tense because I was told by my mother that people who deliver babies through C-Section never get back in shape (it's a myth).

I really got panicked and now when I recall on the same night around 12 AM I got some cramps which just came and went away. I was not sure as I was into labor pain so I never disturbed anyone and just somehow managed with the pain. The due date was still away and even the doctor checked me a day before there was no chance of me going into labor and I really never knew what labor pain feels like. The pain was very intense but it used to come and go away and yes it kept me awake all night. Even though my mother suggested to me that it might be some digestion issues and after trying all medications the pain was there and I went to the doctor where he confirmed yes that was labor pain and my water broke at home only so officially I was into labor 15 days earlier than my due date.

After being in labor pain for almost 24 hours I delivered a baby girl with a birth weight of 4.8 kgs and that too was a normal delivery with lots and lots of struggle and pain. My baby was healthy and beautiful with lots of hair on her head and looked more of a doll with so much hair on her head so the bottom line is everything went well and I came back home with the best gift of my life.

Friends, relatives, neighbors and closed ones to the family were invited to attend the function for celebration of the baby homecoming and yes people came in from far and near just to see her but to my surprise they were much interested in seeing me like how can I look so horrible and how I have gained so much weight and will I ever get back in shape. Everyone present in that party once or maybe twice told me for sure how horrible I looked. My parents kept on defending me by saying that she just had some bad cravings and all this is baby weight and she will soon be back in shape. I never cared about what people had to say as I always believed that what matters is my opinion over anyone else but on that day it literally hit me somewhere.

For the first time in my life I felt bad and that way too bad. I knew this was temporary and I would not always be the same but after everyone looked at me with so many questions made me question my own self. You know it's tough to stay positive when everyone around you is so negative. I was not able to take anymore body shaming so I quickly slipped into my room making an excuse to breastfeed my newborn. I was crying because everyone made me feel so bad at my own party, my parents who were defending me were also at times looking at me as if I am some kind of culprit.

Anyways my husband came to see our child after 7 days as he was travelling due to work. He was overjoyed when he first held her in his arms but he noticed something has changed in me and after asking me many questions he got to know the real reason. He was surprised and shocked that how everyone spoke to me only about weight and why I am getting depressed with it. He told me to not take things very seriously and as I was breastfeeding my daughter he wanted me not to be stressed. He somehow convinced me that once I go back with him we will surely take care of me and my extra weight.

I felt good and I knew he would surely help me and we would together figure something out. So to all the new moms out there, never ever freak out as people need to gossip and this extra weight that you have gained in those nine months will eventually go away but by just over stressing about the things would only make it worse. I have been there, faced with all the criticisms but trust me that should be the last thing on your mind. After giving birth to a new life you should be focused on recovering your body and not on losing weight. You should be concerned about you and your baby's health. Weight gain in pregnancy should be healthy so do keep a check on your food intake and if you are really craving something then have a bite or two just to satisfy your taste buds and try to be physically active.

I would say there are many pregnancy workouts and yogas content available online you can check them or even walking and doing household chores count. Anyways I went back to Delhi to my in-laws where I was actually welcomed with so much love and warmth by my entire family. I came back when my daughter was just a month old and my "weight loss mission" was still on my mind so as soon as I came back I told my husband about my immediate goal though he tried his best to convince me not to focus on that but I was so determined that he finally agreed.

I was obese at that point of time and after delivery eating all those post delivery dry fruits ladoo and foods which are made especially for new moms instead of losing any weight rather I gained more weight so on the day when I first started my weight loss journey I was 112 kgs! Though I was constantly talking about numbers for a very long time, at the same time I was not even feeling good inside. I could barely move and breast feeding my daughter was itself a huge task for me. I was actually on complete bed rest like doing nothing at all apart from taking care of my daughter. I have been a very over protective mother initially and I never gave her to anyone rather I did everything on my own which actually helped me create a great bond with my daughter. But enough was enough and with 112 on the weight loss machine, the time had come to do something about it.

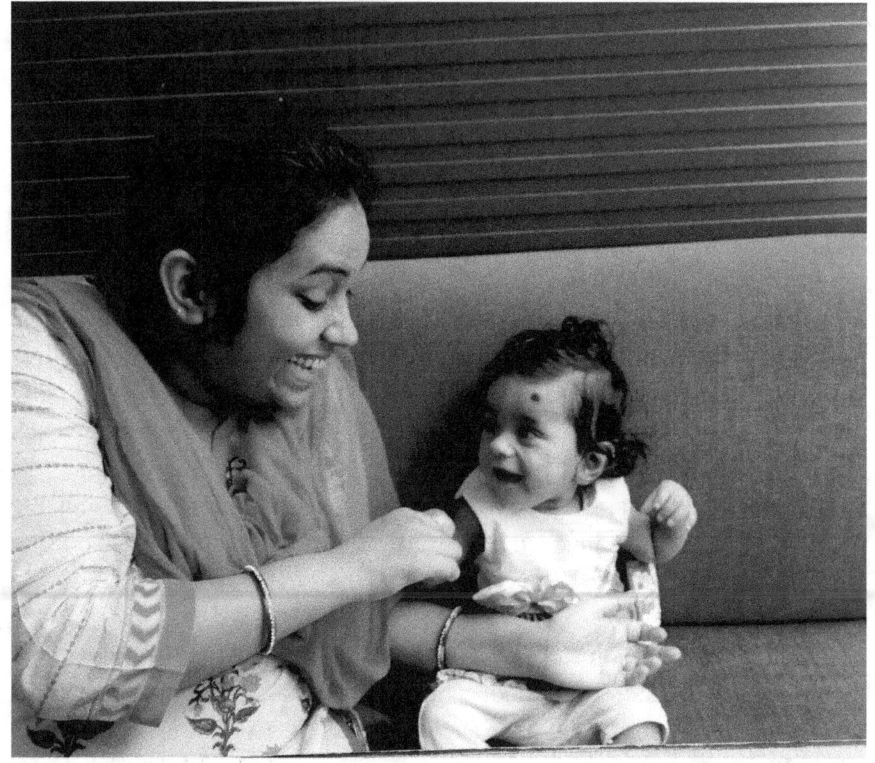

Your dress size doesn't define your happiness.

CHAPTER SEVEN

Mission Weight Loss - Part 1

So after convincing my husband for some time we agreed to visit a dietitian and that too a very famous one. I went and told her my entire story and how I ended up gaining all that extra weight during my pregnancy. She seemed very confident and even told me that this is very natural and just by doing some small changes I will soon be back in shape. I was so happy that I was determined to do everything she recommended and so phase one began. We both went grocery shopping and had a big list to follow which had a lot of food marked as eat and don't eat. If I discuss them all I won't be able to finish it off in one book but anyways to me this was a huge change. There were items which I had never heard of before but as I was very much determined so I followed everything mentioned by her.

I am a big foodie and I have been like this forever though foods have been different at different stages of life but what she has written was not at all like me. I had to start my day with some sort of spice or detox water then after 15 minutes I had to take soaked nuts and then again after 30 mins my breakfast which was so little that I couldn't survive on and felt starved. In the beginning it was great but there was no room for tea, coffee and those dry fruits ladoo which my mother made for me putting in so much love and more than her love was amazing home made ghee.

But anyways I am a person who has got lots of control and discipline, trust me guys I am and if you don't believe me ask my husband he would second that. So her diet consists more of raw veggies and fruits and less of cereals and grains. Previously when I was eating all food prepared at home I was producing loads of milk and sometimes I had to even pump it and dump it as it was way too much but right after following her diet I never had enough milk to even fill my daughter. I was feeling bad but when I told my dietitian about the same she said it's okay and it will get better with time.

Nothing got better, rather my daughter's pediatrician got upset saying that you are playing with your child's health but yes there was progress in weight loss and in a week time I could see the digits coming down though I always felt hungry and cranky and my daughter too lost weight as she was not getting enough milk out of me and she did not like any formulas or powdered milk. I thought losing all those extra weights always brings you some pain and suffering but I had never thought that it would be such a big one.

But now that I know it let me tell you the truth. The truth is that weight loss or fat loss is not at all a painful process and it should not bring any pain or sufferings and if it does then dear you are not doing it right. This is something which I understand now but back then no one ever told me this.

After my daughter's birth I always felt some digestion issues, remember I already told you in the very beginning about my liver problem and how the doctor asked me to get myself checked right after delivery but after becoming a mom I got so busy with my daughter and weight loss mission that I forgot there is something which needed immediate attention. So after 4 months I had some digestion issues and stomach cramps which I completely ignored and never even shared with anyone. But then this happened like after bearing the stomach ache for over a week one night I felt terribly sick. Those stomach cramps got worse and then around 1 AM I started vomiting.

My husband and daughter were asleep and I just never wanted to disturb them so I stayed quiet but when things really got worse and I realised I can't handle the pain anymore, it was around 4 AM when I told my husband to take me to hospital or else I will die. I was in a really bad situation. He immediately took me to the biggest hospital nearby (MAX SUPER SPECIALITY HOSPITAL) and got me admitted to the emergency. My daughter stayed back home though I had to feed her at 5 AM but I had no choice. After running so many tests they came with some loss of vital vitamins that are needed for good liver functioning which led me to this place. As soon as I was admitted they gave me some shots after which I fell asleep and when I woke up it was already noon and my husband was standing right in front of my bed and then I realised he never went back home.

I felt bad because my daughter never knew how to drink from a bottle as she was completely a breast fed child anyways doctors came and explained to my husband how critical the situation is and I am supposed to be admitted for over a week to recover properly. I told them it's not possible as I have a 4 month old baby who is home alone with her grandparents and after convincing them for almost an hour they agreed to discharge me at my own risk and I was strictly told not to breastfeed her. I was also advised not to take any solid meals. You know it was that time when I realised how I ignored my health and my daughters health and how badly it could have ended.

So after thinking a lot about it, **Mission Weight Loss**was aborted for a while.

CHAPTER EIGHT

Mission Weight Loss - Part 2

I believe I had lost a good 10 kgs in 2 month time and then I was asked to focus on my health so I came back to zero now. Life got tough and as no choice was left I started bottle feeding her. Medications went for pretty long and when everything settled down I was back to breastfeeding. This time I wanted to start the process slowly but yes again everything I lost was back again and officially I was 108 kgs on that day. I never spoke to my husband again about it as i knew somewhere he was the one who had suffered a lot along with my daughter so I asked everything from Google & to my surprise Google has answers to all the questions I asked:

How can I lose weight in a week?

How to lose pregnancy weight?

How to lose weight fast?

And so on. Google has answers to all your questions and I am a keen learner so after reading 100+ articles I got to know only one point which is calorie deficit. So as my knowledge grew I could only understand that a calorie deficit is eating less calories than my total daily expenditure of calories and yes for women aged 25-40 this should never be less than 1800 calories as that is the minimum amount of calories our body uses to carry on daily activities. Apart from that I was a breastfeeding mother so after doing all the calculations I reached a number and that was 2200-2400 calories every day.

I belong to an upper middle class family and everything that I own is something my husband and I have really worked hard for. Trust me nothing is gifted or inherited. So while doing all my research work on fitness and weight loss I even had to get back at work as I worked from home and that was something I had to resume again. I can't afford tantrums where someone is doing all the cooking and stuff and I am able to eat every 2 hours. To be honest that is next to impossible and being a mother you have other priorities as well. So I decided to eat homemade food with less oil, no sugar and very less ghee and yes it did help.

Important note: We obsess so much about calories that we forget about our nutritional requirements and foundation of our body. It is important to track your nutritional requirements of the body and if you eat accordingly trust me you will never eat too many calories. Your goal should be eating right from every meal and I will help you to select them.

So I was desperate to lose all that weight which I could see on my body but being desperate doesn't help, rather it creates more problems so instead I decided to go slow. I always made changes and alterations in my diet and never even thought of starting any physical activity. So this time instead of focusing more on weight loss I decided to look after my health and be physically active.

As I used to stay awake the entire night just to feed my daughter so waking up early was a great challenge for me and I never looked at food before eating it but this changed. Waking up early wasn't possible so I started walking during afternoon time when my daughter used to take her afternoon naps. That was the best time to workout and I had a treadmill at home so I started walking easily. Initially it used to make me breathless and I used to have knee pain and the speed used to be 3kmph and that was the maximum effort I was putting in. With time I could see my stamina getting built up and I was able to walk on my own without taking any support so even though I was walking at a speed of 3 still I was happy with my little progress. I saw an ortho doctor for my knee pain and he also suggested to go slow until I lose some weight.

Also I never gave up completely on food. I just started to eat mindfully. I was advised not to have too many oily foods so instead of having those fried dishes I preferred some healthy alternatives and trust me I stopped skipping any of my meals. This process was going very slow but yes I was consistent with it. Tea has always been my weakness and it still is so I never gave up on it completely. Rather, I tried having it post breakfast for at least half an hour. Having tea on an empty stomach is really not good for your overall health. Initially I felt the need to have it soon after waking up but now I was strong enough to control the urges and yes I never had green tea instead of my milk tea. Rather I had a cup of tea with sugar, ginger, cardamom and milk in it.

I knew I don't have to punish myself just to reach a certain dress size and the more I love myself the easier the process would get. I knew my past mistakes and I was not going to repeat them in the future as I have always read everywhere your past is your greatest teacher so never forget your lesson.

CHAPTER NINE

PCOS & How It Changed Me

So I started working out and initially I could notice some changes which really motivated me but after 6 months things were not the same. I could see my weight going up though I did not focus much on the numbers but at the same time my energy levels were going down, my face was getting all hairy and I started to see acne on my face continuously and those were the painful ones. I am not very fond of visiting doctors regularly so I tried plucking those extra hair and even tried some home remedies for acne but everyday it was getting worse. I thought maybe it's just because I am feeding my child but I found it alarming when my periods got irregular and whenever it came it was very painful and then I decided to visit my gynaecologist.

She got some tests done and later told me that I was suffering from PCOS (Polycystic Ovarian Syndrome). I was really not aware what exactly she was talking about and I had never heard of this disease before so she told me about it. While PCOS itself is not life threatening, those who have it are at higher risk for other more serious conditions such as Type II diabetes, cardiovascular problems, endometrial cancer, liver inflammation and some more. There are four types of PCOS: Insulin-resistant PCOS, Inflammatory PCOS, Hidden-cause PCOS, and Pill-induced PCOS. This is the most common type of PCOS.

So for people like me the easiest way to understand it is actually "Hormonal Imbalance" wherein some male hormones increase and that helps you grow those beard like hair on your face. I asked her about medications and yes she did give me a few but at the same time she asked me to maintain a healthy lifestyle in case I don't want to face any more problems. After going through many blood tests, sonography and some more tests landed us to a place where she told me to either I go on medications for my lifetime as you have a diabetes family history from both of your parents or you can control it by maintaining a good and healthy lifestyle.

That was the game changer and on the very same day I decided that enough is enough and I am not letting myself suffer just because I made some wrong choices for my body. You know what is more important: your mental shift once you decide you have to move forward there is no going back and the same was with me. I had decided that I am going to treat myself the way I want others to treat me with the same love and respect. I am sharing a picture where you can see those flared acne on my cheeks which were very painful and hair all over my face.

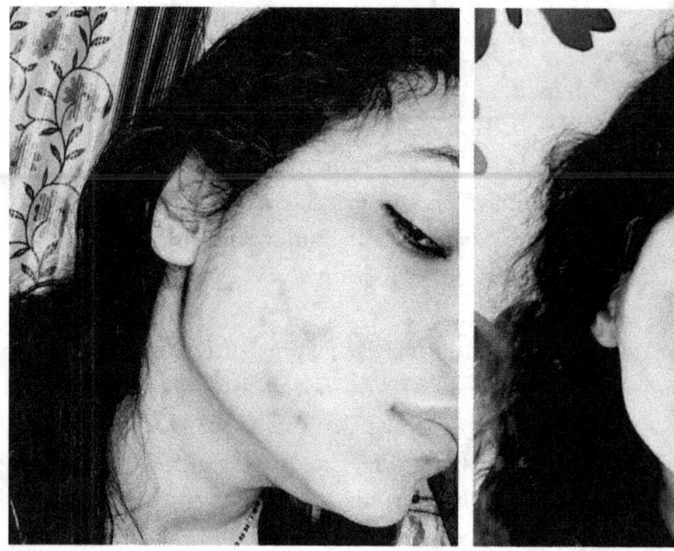
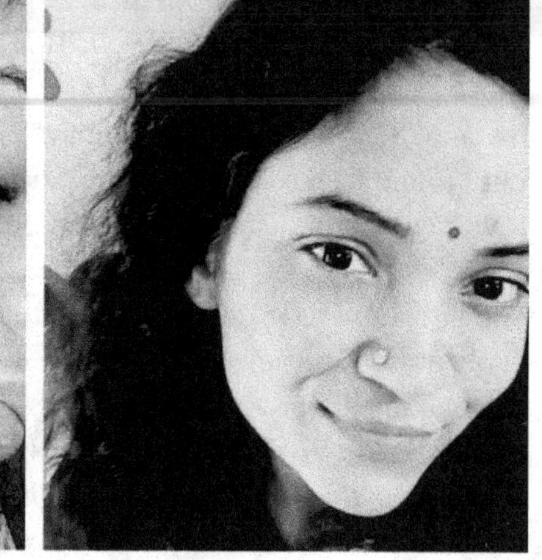

Before & After PCOS

Dermatologist suggested that I should go for laser hair removal and yes I did try but it didn't take me anywhere as those hairs kept coming back so I tried a much cheaper and painless way of removing them by using a face epilator and it is very handy and cost effective. It's up to you guys what you think is best for you so go for that.

My Daily Routine After I Was Diagnosed With PCOS

I started my day with a morning walk and yoga at home. I learned yoga online and I never forced myself into anything. I took my time to learn it and yes it helped me to become more flexible and at the same time, also helped me to calm myself as I was also doing meditation along with yoga. We all believe that we need to huff and puff and to sweat like anything to lose weight but trust me I never did anything as such and still lost weight and got my hormones in check so yoga helps. There is a misconception that you don't lose weight with yoga but it's all a myth. Weight loss with yoga is very much possible and is also effective in maintaining strength and flexibility of your own body. It not only makes you look good from outside rather it helps you achieve that inner peace in your mind. Remember any sort of physical activity is good so do what you are comfortable with.

I knew it would take some time and I was not in a hurry. I decided to go easy on myself and do it more patiently. You know everyone talks so much about exercise on the internet but people who are beginners or have gained way too much really need a start point and it is really difficult to find that point. I have been with the fitness industry during my teen years and I know how to start so even though it looked really tough still I decided to start so treadmill did wonders to me. I was obese so walking at a stretch of 15 minutes was way too much for me but slowly with time I was able to walk for a long time and with time I was able to walk at a much better pace. I am not asking you to buy a treadmill (a big NO) but as I was living in the National capital of our country and really never had a big garden close to our place or a private terrace so that is the best I could do. I even had to take care of my daughter and her noon nap time was never fixed so I had to adjust my time accordingly.

PCOS doesn't go away completely but yes it gets in control and as I have seen myself losing all those extra weight and getting that acne free face I was sure my hormones are much balanced now. There is not a single mark on my face and the hair which was there is still there but now there is no new hair growth can be seen and above all my periods are regular with less pain as I always had pain since it started so no extra pain now. The diagnosis of PCOS made me more mindful of my body and what it needs so it was a blessing in disguise.

CHAPTER TEN

It Gets Better With Time

As it is said once you start seeing the result you crave more of it and the same happened with me. With each passing day I was feeling more strong and yes every progress is a progress even though how big or small it is. Be your own best friend and treat yourself always the way you want others to treat you. If you are able to do anything better than yesterday then it is a progress so always be proud of yourself and appreciate your effort. Always try to be 1% better than yesterday and then you are on the right track.

One thing I got rid of this time was the weighing scale because I believe it just gives you the number and keeps you into that spiral where if you don't see the change in number you tend to give up easily and I realised it's not helping in my journey and I found a different way of tracking my progress so I shifted myself to clicking progress pics talking of which I used to click one picture every week in the same position in the same set of clothes and in a month itself I had 4 pictures in the same position to see the difference. The number on the scale never changed but my body did. I was not doing any sort of xyz or yoyo diets so I never saw any drastic changes in my body but yes I did notice some small changes and those were the initial milestones which I achieved.

With every passing day I realised my body started feeling better. I was sleeping well, eating well and was feeling more energetic and moreover my skin looked flawless. I just made some small changes but I saw great results and that helped me and motivated me a lot. Always remember you don't need anyone else to motivate you, you are your own motivation and stop looking out at others to motivate you.

Never compare yourself to others because you are the creator of your own life and happiness so don't destroy it. When you look at others you feel so convinced that they own everything that you have dreamt of like that dream house, dream body, dream car, dream relationships and so on but you know while looking at others you are just devaluing yourself and doing self deprecating talks which tells your subconscious mind that you are worthless and doesn't stand anywhere so stop doing that. Instead of looking at others it's better to work on your own self growth and if you really have to compare then compare your today to your yesterday and see how you have made it much better and enjoy it.

So after walking continuously and building up an exercise regimen for 6 months I decided to join a gym as I wanted to start my workout under some expert supervision. As my husband saw my dedication and will power he got me the membership of Fitness First Select City Walk along with a good personal trainer. You know nothing comes free and this membership was worth it anyways so I started my journey with a fantastic trainer who helped me in the best ways possible. I wanted to do strength training as I thought it's really time to tone up myself.

As I was doing it after a long time, lifting weights was not an easy task. I used to give up very easily but she kept pushing me and so within months I could say I got better with weights and yes of course people who really want to know about the numbers during my weight loss journey the number on the scale showed 80 kgs when I joined. I used to workout with her like everyday for an hour and post strength training I used to do some Zumba or any sort of Cardio.

Always remember while doing weight training your focus should not be on the amount of weight you are lifting rather your focus should always be on the form and remember your form should never suffer. Don't lift weights to show off or to do an ego boost rather lift weight as much as your body allows you to and be perfect with your form. What I am going to say may or may not make any sense to you all but anyhow I will express my view, You really don't need a gym or fitness club membership to get back in shape. Yes I am a gym lover but actually I don't love the gym.

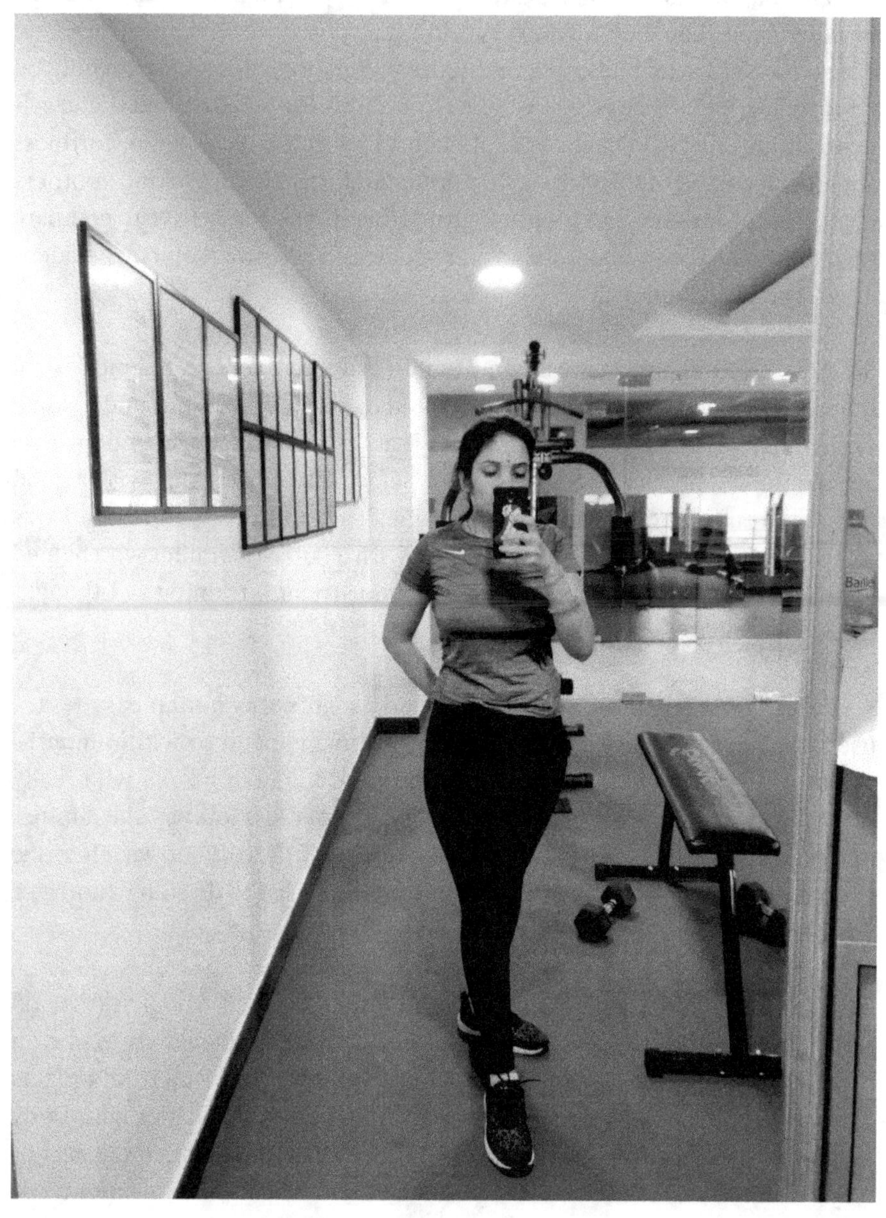

Staying Consistent Is The Key

I love working out and trying new and different exercises which can be performed out there. If you can't afford it don't even think about it you can do it with/without gym all you need is your body and will power. I joined the gym because I really wanted someone to help me learn all the forms and how to target different muscle groups and now that I have learnt so much I can do my workouts anytime, anywhere and yes I love weights so I have invested some good amount of money in dumbbells. In case you can't invest in a home gym remember your body itself is capable of everything. You can do so many body weight exercises, circuits, HIIT, Yoga, pilates which require no weights and they are the best workouts.

So I have been talking a long about exercise and physical activity till now. Let me tell you something about my eating habits as well. As it is said that abs are made in the kitchen and so I agree with it. If you really want to lose weight or get back in shape or maintain a healthy lifestyle you really need to see what's on your plate though I agree food is not a rocket science.

During my fitness journey I just made sure that I ate right every two hours without starving myself and till date I never followed any sort of fancy diet. I never switched to any health drinks, shakes, weight loss tea, detox drinks or any sort of juices just to lose some extra kilos. Remember, it gets better with time so just stick to a healthy lifestyle and you will be at your best for sure real soon.

CHAPTER ELEVEN

Nutrition & Weight Loss

To me simplicity is the key to being healthy and fit and I personally believe that simpler the better. Previously I never had any knowledge on food and nutrition but with time I learnt a lot. I even enrolled myself into a nutrition course just to understand the benefit of food and it's role in our life. I realised how undervalued nutrition is and how we sometimes fail to understand food as a source of nutrition to our body. We are so lost in today's world and copying others that we really fail to understand what exactly our body needs and how we can nourish it. Looking at food just in terms of calories is not at all helpful. Food is more than protein, carbohydrates, minerals and vitamins, if you are eating right you will lead a healthy life. You all will be surprised to know that food plays a major role in various diseases.

It is usually said that if you spend more calories than you consume you are into calorie deficit which makes you lose weight but always remember that our body has to function daily and every second while we are breathing and for that also you need energy so just don't think that you should consume calories what you burn through exercise but practically we are so much into fast/junk food these days that we just look into the calories and not into the nutritional value of the food.

Calories are different for different food groups and let me explain it to you in a much simpler way. An apple which has 100 calorie also contains fibre which does not let it digest quickly, contains different forms of vitamins, folic acid and does not spike your blood sugar levels instantly and also keeps you full for some time, it is not processed or packaged hence full of goodness and the best part is you can have it anytime anywhere. On the other hand, a glass of soda which also has 100 calories has no fibre in it, can be digested easily, spikes your blood sugar level, has no vitamins in it and is harmful for you and your overall health. Both of these foods are the same when it comes to calories but their nutritional values are way too different. Apples which are healthy have got the goodness of nature on the other hand any soda which also has the same calories does more harm than good.

Everyone talks so much about sugar and now they have created many alternatives that they are using in the place of sugar. Trust me one or two tablespoons of sugar is not as dangerous as the ones you are having in your fast foods or diet sodas. Hidden sugars are more dangerous than the one which we eat or drink intentionally because you know at least how much sugar you ate or drank.

Weight loss industry is growing everyday and it is mainly growing on our weakness. Just because we believe sodas contain blank sugar so we switched to diet sodas without even thinking once, because we think biscuits, chips, cookies are bad now we switched to sugar free biscuits, baked chips and so on. Logically we are just swapping from one unhealthy food item to another believing it's all good. What we need to understand is we don't need sodas or biscuits and if we do want to eat it, let it be the normal one.

I am not against any product or brand but while studying nutrition I realised how we are making fools of ourselves. This is why I insist on making it simple, I just follow the sun and yes I am not a fan of junk food anymore. There are people who want to gain weight but remember there is a key to it. Healthy or unhealthy weight gain. People who are looking to gain weight in a healthy way are the ones who are looking forward to increasing their muscle mass not the fat percentage while others who are looking to do it in an unhealthy way like eating all junk are going to increase their body fat.

Whether it's weight gain or weight loss it should always be done in a healthy way and that is why I never support any crash diet. Crash diets might look good but they never help you in the long run and I believe in a sustainable diet (something which you can do for the rest of your life). Fad diets are like those toxic relationships which makes you feel so good in the beginning, gives you butterflies in the stomach but when it goes away it leaves you with so much darkness, you lose your complete identity and it makes you question your own worth. In the same way when you go for crash diets you initially lose some water weight but with time you become weak, you start losing hair, your skin looks dull and pale, you can't sleep, you are not able to carry on your daily activities properly so choose wisely when it comes to diet and relationships. Choose only those which can last forever.

If you believe you can live without food for the rest of your life then you should surely go on such diets because personally I can't do this. These diets will not only take the body fat but your muscle mass as well and your body will start losing all it's necessary components and down the line in the future instead of flaunting that body you will lose that glow on your face, those hair on your head and above all your strength and energy would be way too less and you will always feel irritated and cranky. If you don't enjoy the process you should not do it. We should always try to eat a balanced meal and once a week you can have your favourite cheat meal.

I don't go for cheat days, rather I prefer eating a cheat meal. You know it's okay to have a 500 calorie deficit everyday but going too low on calories can actually cause more harm to your body . To achieve a good and faster metabolism you need to eat at regular intervals and that too you should eat right. Food is the fuel for your body and it is up to you what kind of fuel you chose to put in. I have seen youngsters playing much with the calorie game but as soon as they start crossing their 30 they are the one complaining more of knee problems, back problems and joint problems. Their posture suffers and they are the one suffering different kinds of diseases so if you are really not interested in going down that lane it's better if you start making changes in your early life.

I have always had the benefit of eating home cooked food and today also I prefer making meals at home. Why home cooked meals are considered healthy and nutritious? First of all when someone cooks at home they cook it with love and when you love someone you take care of every minute detail, like not using too much oil, salt or spices, using fresh vegetables, cleaning and maintaining hygiene throughout the cooking process and above all serving it hot and fresh. I know the difference between the food when it comes out of the kitchen and when it comes out of a packet. In my weight loss journey I looked at my food as fuel and I enjoyed each and every meal.

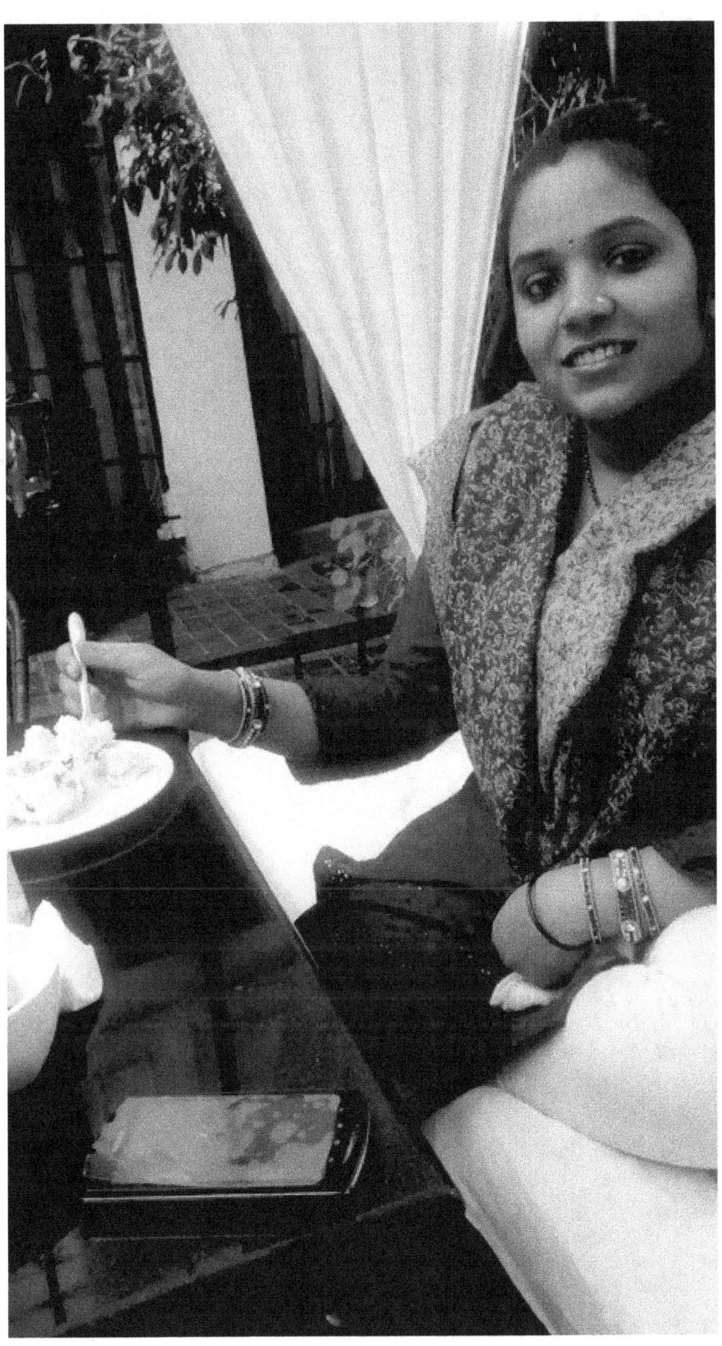

Me enjoying my food guilt free

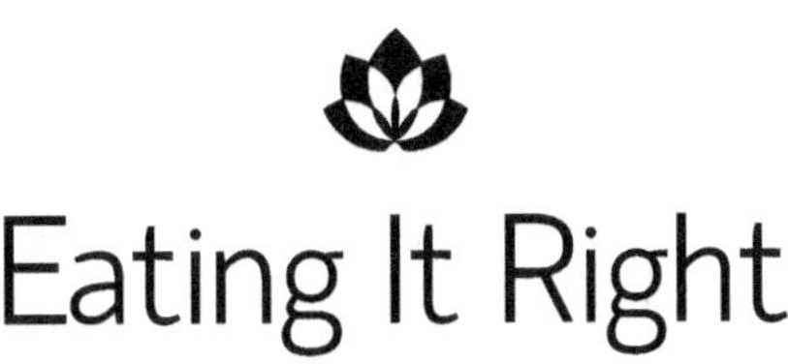

Eating It Right

There is a famous myth that vegetarians don't get enough protein from their food, even at one point of time even I believed it too and so they should always have some sort of protein shakes as a protein supplement. To be honest, a vegetarian diet also has a large supply of protein but if you prefer to take some whey protein for muscle repair or maintenance that is also not bad. Being a vegetarian I know my options and I prefer using them instead of going for any supplement. I have tried some protein powder but it doesn't suit me so I tried increasing my protein intake through my food. Different forms of lentils, chickpeas, paneer, tofu, cheese and so many things are there to use as protein supplements.

Speaking of my diet, I follow the sun religiously like as soon as I wake up I drink two glasses of plain water or lukewarm water and after 15 minutes I have my soaked dry fruits like 4 almonds, 4 raisins or munakka along with 2 soaked walnuts. After an hour I have my breakfast which is the biggest meal of the day for me. It usually have a fruit, I go with any local seasonal fruit then a plate of poha, upma, oats porridge, cauliflower stuffed roti with ghee, vegetable stuffed roti or paratha, paneer stuffed paratha or for that matter I would say any paratha along with some curd or home made chutney such as mint coriander or gooseberry chutney.

After half an hour post breakfast I have a cup of tea and that too with milk and sugar. Around 11 AM I take any snack. Sometimes it's a sandwich or buttermilk or anything like banana, grilled sweet potato or whatever is easily available at home. My lunch is usually around 1 PM in which I eat rice and lentil along with some vegetable curry, pickle, a chapati and some freshly cut salads. I eat a wholesome lunch and I eat it very slowly like enjoying every bit of it.

My evening snack compromise of some nuts and a cup of tea and my dinner is around 8 PM as I sleep around 12AM and I don't want to indulge in any night time snacking so I prefer to eat around 8 and that consists of any vegetable curry along with some lentils and 2 chapatis. I eat regular white rice though the quantity is pretty less but I don't like the taste of brown rice and I stick to 100% whole wheat flour and I even switch to jowar, bajra or multigrain chapati as well because I don't want to irritate my digestive system so I don't try any sort of low carb flour or keto flour.

The most important thing I forgot to mention is that my plate contains ghee in almost every meal and that ghee is homemade by me. I don't trust any brand and so I prefer making ghee at home safely and maintaining all kinds of hygiene. I would actually love to share the recipe with you all for the same though it's very simple and you can find it on YouTube or Google.

Before I dig any deeper into ghee or it's recipe let me tell you all that all fats aren't bad and not taking bad fat doesn't mean that you switch yourself completely to a fat free diet or liquid diet which includes soups, salads and juices. According to studies, mono unsaturated fats and poly unsaturated fats are known as the "good fats" because they are good for your heart, your cholesterol, and your overall health. These fats can help to lower the risk of heart disease and stroke, lower bad LDL cholesterol levels, while increasing good HDL. There are two types of fat that should be eaten sparingly: saturated and trans fatty acids. Both can raise cholesterol levels, clog arteries, and increase the risk for heart disease.

To be more specific about it, stop eating junk foods and processed foods as they are high in trans fat and are the most unhealthy ones. Whenever you buy something just check the nutritional value of the product by looking at the back of it and you would be able to see the nutritional information about the product. So maybe while eating just a packet of chips or for that matter anything you really don't know what harm you are causing to yourself.

When it comes to ghee it's all natural and doesn't contain preservatives or trans fat. It is a rich source of antioxidants and also helps to fight against cancer. Though it is a storehouse of fat but don't get stressed as it only contain the healthy ones monounsaturated omega 3s. So adding ghee to your diet would not only make your meal healthy and tasty but will also help your body to get its nourishment.

To all of you who eat non vegetarian foods let me tell you no food is bad and you can always include fish, eggs, chicken or any sort of meat products in your diet just try to make it less oily like not frying it too much and you can take in lesser quantity, you can also eat grilled form of meat with some salads and rice with it as it will be a complete meal and is also very healthy as it is a complete balanced meal.

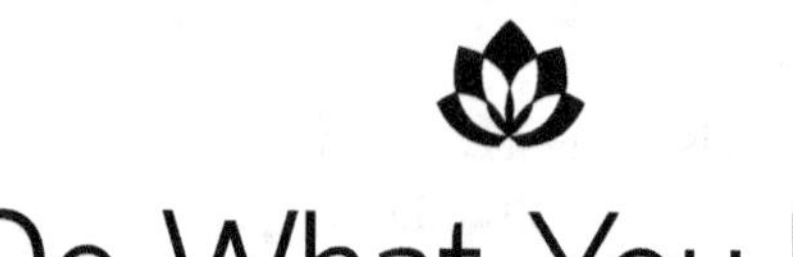

CHAPTER THIRTEEN

Do What You Love

Weight loss industry has created so much panic among us that whenever we hear the word "Diet", we believe that we need to starve all day and eat all unflavoured and tasteless food. This isn't true while many still follow those crash diets but that is not sustainable and that is something which falls in the unhealthy group. I believe that the weight loss/ fat loss process should be slow but it should take you a long way and of course you should enjoy this process.

I always believe that you should always do what you love or else you won't be able to continue doing it for the rest of your life. As I already spoke the word love once so let me just elaborate on it. You know if you don't love yourself you can't do anything right with yourself. I will seriously write a complete book on self love but let me just talk a little about it. You know self love is not about visiting a salon every other day or buying expensive jewellery or doing anything just to show others that you care about yourself. Actually it's a lot more than that and this is a topic which is never talked about. It's great to look a certain way and wear your favourite dress but you know what is more needed is to accept yourself the way you are.

You don't need anyone to validate this for you, you don't need anyone to complete you. You complete yourself and no one is you so that is your superpower. The moment you realise your own self worth and accept your own body you don't think of punishing it. Just by doing some crash diets or going on some juice diets not only weakens your immune system but also makes your metabolism slow.

You need to understand that the weight you have gained hasn't come overnight so you just can't lose it in a week. Don't fall for those promising ads which lure you by saying that just by drinking some health shakes as meal replacement would help you shed off all those extra pounds. Respect your body just because last night you ate too much doesn't mean that you have to kill your self next day in the gym or starve yourself to balance those calories. Your body needs love not hate so respect your body and instead of obsessing about weight loss focus more on being healthy and staying fit.

Ditch that weighing scale which shows you some number and reminds you that you still need to lose some more numbers, your body changes everyday and keeping some number as a goal weight in your mind makes things go bad. If you really want to track the progress, keep track of your progress pics and I believe when you start eating well you can see an overall change like you feel energetic throughout the day, your hair doesn't fall out in lumps, your skin glows, you sleep well, you don't feel bloated. I know most of you must be thinking that as I have lost my excess weight that is why I am giving this sort of tips but trust me I have been there I have felt the same thing and whenever someone spoke to me about eating foods at regular intervals I also hated it but now I understand it and I love this process.

The never ending weight loss cycle is very dangerous. You lose it by doing some crazy diet but as soon as you start eating food again you gain it all back, you feel lethargic all day, there are lots of cravings and you don't get enough energy to exercise well, your face looks dull, your hair falls out and you age very rapidly. This is an unending cycle and it goes on forever so if you really want to invite some major health problems you can try this crash diet, juice diets or detox weight loss.

I know it's easier said than done but trust me guys I have been there and after trying all stupid and crazy diets supported and promoted by others I have faced all the consequences and I really don't want any of you to go through this. Trust me you can eat anything just remember the quantity and of course the timing. These days we all are so scared of food that the instant we think of it we only connect it with calories and weight gain. Food has a major role apart from those calories and weight gain. We should be more focused on micros and macros instead of calories.

Okay now I have used one more term which most of you are not even aware of and as I have already used the term so let me elaborate it for you. Actually macros and micros are the foods that we should look at while nourishing your body. People talk so much about carbohydrates, proteins and fats but we mostly miss on some more terms such as vitamins, minerals and amino acids. Food is the only source of fuel and the fuel we chose for our body is what gives us the result. If you own a petrol car you surely can't expect it to run on diesel and of course you won't even try because this is what you have paid your hard earned money for. We human beings mostly focus on material things that we pay for instead of looking after our health which is our only wealth. Don't you think if you stay healthy and happy you can perform better and for a longer period of time. So if you would not prefer to fuel your car with wrong fuel, why would you do the same for your own body?

Let me put one more example just to make myself more clear. Can you run your car without any fuel in it? I know you all would say of course not how stupid this question is. This is what we should expect from our body as well. You cannot starve yourself and expect your body to perform amazingly and function properly. Use the right food, choose the right one and eat accordingly. You don't need to starve yourself just because you want to achieve a certain shape or size. Your body doesn't need calories just to perform some exercises. Its major need for calories is to perform all bodily functions along with exercise. Your body burns only 30% of the calorie through exercise rest is used by the body to perform its functions and carry on its daily activities.

Nowadays so many diets are in the market that people usually get confused to choose which one to go along with. Fact is always choose the food which you have been eating since your childhood and learn to eat local and seasonal. First of all it's very pocket friendly and secondly it hasn't travelled much so it will be fresh and the amount of preservatives will be quite less.

My job here is not to stop you from trying anything new but I just want you all to remember what exactly you had through your childhood and even after eating your favorite meals regularly without any guilt you were still thin and never had any medical issues. Your waist size was too perfect and your skin glowed without any skin regimen and of course you just applied coconut oil on your hair and nothing else. We never had any problems falling asleep, we never suffered anxiety and we never went to any salon or doctors. Just because I was going to a gym doesn't mean you can't lose weight at home.

I am writing this book in pandemic and trust me I have not been to the gym since March 2020 and I am still working out at the comfort of my time at my own pace and I am doing great. I am getting confident in my own skin and if you want you can check my instagram handle where I share my stories daily as a part of motivation like how you can also use your bodyweight and train yourself.

This is all a mind game and you just need little motivation to keep yourself going. There is nothing like rocket science to understand your own body. If you are not comfortable in exercising like people who are beginners or are obese may not feel motivated enough to exercise then start walking. If you don't want to go out for any reason, just walk inside your house continuously and if you have an independent house just walk up and down the stairs or you can start with yoga and pilates they are great to strengthen your body and will also help you to establish a mind-body connection. Just don't hurry the process and start with like 5 surya namaskars and do it continuously for 15 days when you feel good and get used to it, simply increase it to 10 and so on.

There is no limit to it and you can do it as much as you want. Looking at social media for inspiration wont help because the pictures and videos that you see on social media are of fitness models who have trained their bodies for many years to look like that and they are being paid to show off and their diet is not something you can follow. Moreover, always be realistic when it comes to your dream body. You should not focus on numbers, rather focus on how good your body feels.

CHAPTER FOURTEEN

Connect Mind With Body

I heard many times about mind-body connections and how useful it is if you are really trying to get healthy but I never had one. In all these years one thing I learnt was if you really want to lose weight you need to know your own body and respect it. There is lots of biochemistry involved in the human body and I believe we should atleast have the idea of it because when you don't know enough about your own body how could you expect that you will treat it right. We all human beings have the same body anatomy but there is lots of difference between males and females. We all are different individuals and so are our needs as we don't have the same eating pattern sleeping pattern or we don't even carry out the same physical activities.

Every food we eat or for that matter every calorie we consume is not burnt only through exercise or physical activity. There are calories which are required for a human body to carry on its basic activities even when you are leading a completely sedentary lifestyle. So thinking all the time that you should eat less calories just because you are carrying on a sedentary lifestyle or you are not exercising enough doesn't help every organ in your body. It requires a certain amount of calories to work and food is the only way through which we provide nutrition and energy to our body.

Now let me talk about exercise now. While it is good to stay physically active and exercising is our major need but remember over exercising or under exercising is not good, so make sure that you are exercising in a good way and it has to be quality. Exercising 4-5 times a week for 45 minutes to an hour is enough and if you have been exercising for quite some time then you should train all muscle groups, just remember do not train the same muscle group in the next 24-48 hours as our muscles need time to repair and maintain. While learning nutrition I realised that our body is not just made up of food it is 70% water and so never ignore the fact that liquid is necessary so drink as much water as you can but that does not mean you will start drinking 10 L of water everyday, just enough so approx 4-5 L.

Did you know that eating less can be harmful? In our body there is a hormone known as leptin which is responsible for the fat loss of the body. But let me tell you how this hormone works. It does not work if you eat way too less calorie because if you eat too less calorie then it gets shocked and doesn't allow you to lose fat rather it tries to store fat as a form of storage as it expect you won't provide body enough energy. That is why it is said that everyone should eat a cheat meal once in a week guilt free so that leptin hormone doesn't drop and keeps working fine and your metabolism stays up and running.

Now you must be thinking what is the exact calorie that we should eat in order to maintain a daily healthy lifestyle so the exact number of calories for a woman who is not physically active and is leading a sedentary lifestyle is 1800 calories and for a man who is not physically active and is leading a sedentary lifestyle is 2400 calories and let me tell you these are for young people. Now there are people who think that in order to have 1800 calories or 2400 calories in your body you can opt for any food which is actually not true. It's not only calories that matters but what matters the most is nutrition. If the nutritional value of your body is not met then eating food which is high in calories would only increase the fat storage in your body which in the long-term would cause you various ailments and diseases along with weight gain or your skin will become loose and saggy.

CHAPTER FIFTEEN

Food & Healthy Lifestyle

Food is a very huge topic which needs to be discussed properly and through my next book I am planning to do a detailed work on food and exercise which will share in-depth knowledge about these two topics. I wish I could have known so much about fitness, food and exercise in my early 20s then I could have been altogether a different person. But it's never too late and irrespective of how you felt yesterday has nothing to do with your tomorrow. You can always stand up and change the story all by yourself.

Remember you are not losing those extra kgs just because you want to fit into some xyz dress rather you want to lose all those extra fat so that you can lead a healthy life throughout and fitness is not a destination, it's a lifetime journey which never ends. If you look at yourself in the mirror and you find that there is still a 1% chance of improvement then go ahead and do it. It's now or never and especially for all those women out there who are reading this you are the one who is inspiring your own family (specially your kids). We love our family unconditionally but what we forget is that we need to love ourselves first and when we are healthy and happy then only we can extend the same vibe around us.

I can easily tell you when I initially started my weight loss journey it was all about losing my pregnancy and post pregnancy fat but it took me no time to realise that it's more about consistency and commitment. Being a mother of a daughter I know my priorities have changed and I need to invest more time in her but at the same time we all get 24 hours a day and how we choose to spend our entire day completely depends on us. I was never a morning person but now I wake up early in the morning and spend most of my time doing yoga or I go out for a walk/run.

With every passing day I am really getting more concerned about food around us. Most of us nowadays rely on packed food as first of all it is easily available and secondly it's way too convenient to eat. I would say a big NO to everything which comes out of a packet. If given a choice I would prefer to even get oils fresh too which is really not possible but yes at least I am not a big fan of packed foods even not for kids at any age. In our early years when packed foods weren't there we had only fresh home made or market snacks which was still a better option than these packed stuff. If you don't have time to cook, plan your meals ahead and try to shop for a week before so that you have all your supplies with you whenever you want to cook.

I work from home and I am the one cooking as well so I plan my meals ahead and it is very easy to cook when you have a clear idea of what will be served next day on the plate. I am working towards my fitness and health but that doesn't mean that the entire family won't eat what I eat. So I have planned my meal accordingly and people who say that diet foods are bland are not even aware that you don't have to take taste out of the food just to get healthy. You can get healthy by eating right, not by eating tasteless food.

I have been there giving all the possible excuses to myself for not losing weight but at the end of the day I realised it's not anything else that is creating a problem, it's my own mindset which is the one causing all the troubles. There is nothing called bloating if you are hydrating enough, not eating packed high sodium foods and sleeping right. Here sleeping right doesn't mean closing your eyes and thinking about all the foods you can eat or thinking about anything but not sleeping, sleeping actually means taking a proper nap for straight 8-9 hours and to have a good night sleep you need to eat right food. There is no detox diet or detox juice available which will cleanse your body and stomach.

You are exactly what you eat, so instead of buying those foods which say about quick detox or weight loss try eating something that is local and pocket friendly. Just because bananas are cheap and detox juice is expensive doesn't mean that is something you should opt for. Look for food which is not only easy on your pocket but also known to your stomach and if we could have survived on juices then why are we blessed with teeths and a tongue with so much saliva? Applying common sense in daily life and food choices both will be easier for you. Just because a celebrity is endorsing some brand of oil or product doesn't mean that you need to buy that one even though he/she is your favorite one. I know it's easy to get impressed and flattered after seeing such ads but after studying and doing my research work for a long time now I realise that celebrities are being paid a hefty amount of cash to endorse so and so product and of course you don't have to put your hard earned money into it because they are not using it either.

Do you think they have time to shop for their oils, soap and shampoos? No, they have got a lot on their plate. Trust me I don't think that they don't even know which oil is being used in their kitchen by their cook or chef. I have nothing against anyone, it's their job to do and it's our job to understand what works best for us. If you can afford it then of course try anything you want but your body isn't a lab where you should be experimenting.

CHAPTER SIXTEEN

Starting Your Weight Loss Journey

Please understand that weight loss isn't so complicated and you also don't try to complicate things. If you really want to start on your fitness journey try with these things first.

Start With 5000 Steps Daily

Now there are many smart/fitness watches available in the market which you can easily use and if you can't afford any just try to install any app like pedometer and try using it to get an idea of your steps. Start with 5K steps and gradually keep increasing it and with time you will see the difference.

Use A Smaller Plate

Initially when you want to start your weight loss journey you really need to be patient and take one step at a time. Go with your regular meals but just shrink down the size of your plate and of your meal too and with time you will realise how much food you actually need to fill your stomach. For example, start with one chapati and some rice along with dal, curry, curd for your lunch. If you feel full it's great but in case you still feel hungry add half a chapati more, don't just go ahead and take one whole. First take half and then still you want then only take the other half.

Plan Your Meals

Planning your meal in advance is a great way to start because this is the only way you can see your entire week and can realise where you went wrong. We keep taking surplus calories when we don't plan our meals in advance. You need to make a complete plan including your snacks too and don't forget to add your tea and coffee.

Hydrate Yourself

This is something we all know but we all ignore, water is 70% of our body but that is something we underestimate. If you really want to know about a detox drink then it's water and you can have 5 litres of water a day and yes don't drink too much as it may impact your organs and you can land up in the ER.

Start Some Exercise

Walking is staying physically active and it is not considered as exercise while running, sprinting or jogging is considered as they make your heart beat faster and you really have to keep your pace up but if you are really new to fitness and is not comfortable exercising then start walking and you can also add some sort of yoga as well.

Get Your Routine Blood Tests Done

In case you eat well, exercise 4-5 times a week and lead a good physical and emotional life but still you are gaining too much weight and are suffering mood swings it's good to get a blood profile done and to test if you have any underlying cause for the same.

Eat Your Dinner Early

This is a habit which hinders your weight loss process and until and unless you are not someone who is working too late at night or has some reasons due to which you are forced to eat late at night then it's something you can't help or else try to eat your dinner at least 2 hours before bedtime and if possible walk for at least half an hour post dinner that would help the digestion process and evening walks helps with good night sleep too.

Ditch The Weighing Scale

If you are one of those who keep checking your weight every other morning then I would say stop as this is not healthy. Your weight machine only shows a number which not only tells about fat but it also includes muscle mass, water weight and other components as well. If you really want to check your progress then compare in terms of your health, your dress size, how you feel and of course how you sleep. If these changes are good then you are on the right track and numbers never tell you how strong you are or how far you have come.

Try To Take Rest & Good Sleep

While exercising is important and so is rest, never ever underestimate the power of rest. Working out is good but you need to rest so that you can perform well again the next day so to perform better you need to let your body rest and recover. Training thrice or four times a week is good to start with but don't drag your body for hours. If it is asking for rest then you need to stop and allow yourself to rest.

Love & Accept Yourself

No two bodies are the same and so are the sizes. When I go lean my upper body shrinks completely while my lower body still looks heavy and strong and there are girls whose glutes are way too lean. Comparing my body to someone else only brings me pain and discomfort. I have compared myself to others all the time but since I realised my body is unique and my happiness is not anyhow associated with my size my thoughts about me have completely changed. Now I feel much better in my own skin and I really love my mermaid figure. So it's you who has to accept your own self irrespective of how others treat you. Body shaming is something we all have to suffer, especially people who are fat but it should not impact your mental and emotional state, if you love the way you are it doesn't matter what others think of you. Loving and accepting yourself is way beyond weight loss and it requires lots of time and effort to fall in love with your own self. I know it takes lots of patience to fall in love with your ownself, I have been put through body shaming many a times just because I was obese and out of size but there are people who are obese not by choice or unhealthy lifestyle or poor eating habits but due to some underlying medical cause/issues. So if you are trying your best and still your body is heavy then its okay to accept that and stay healthy. Distance yourself away from people who tie your value to a certain dress size. Your aim should be to remain healthy and fit.

Be Patient

If you really want to continue the journey you need to be patient just because something works for me right away in a span of a few months it doesn't mean that it would work in the same way for you like I said we all have different bodies and they behave differently. So what works for me may not at all work for you and what works for you won't work for me. It's simple to understand your own body for which you really need to invest a lot of time and you have to be patient throughout your journey. Just to get rid of those extra weight don't think of trying some calorie deficit diet like opting for any juice diet that is not a good option only for your metabolism but also in the long run you would be inviting more health problems. If you want to lose weight then I would say it's easy to lose weight but it's way too tough to maintain the same weight that you have lost and of course you don't want to gain back more than what you lost so instead of looking for short-term goals it's best to think of the long run. Being patient not only helps you get rid of those extra kgs but would also help you to maintain a good metabolism and you won't look sick.

Click Pictures

When I say ditch the weighing scale people usually ask me then how I should check my progress. To check your progress the best way is to keep clicking pictures. Every week take one picture of yours on an empty stomach and keep doing it. It's better if you take a complete picture with less clothes or tight clothes in front of a mirror. Keep doing it for a span of 6 months and then notice the changes. I bet if you are doing everything right then you will surely see a huge change.

Progress Takes Time

If you are not a beginner and are already on your weight loss journey then I would say that keep going and if in case you have hit a plateau then look after your diet and exercise as maybe you are doing something wrong somewhere. You should not give up irrespective of how tough it seems. If you keep working out and eating right then of course you will see the change. Remember progress takes time and where you are today is not because you went wrong or led a wrong lifestyle just for a few days. So don't lose heart, progress is happening and you are getting better.

Consistency Is The Key

While I believe fitness is a lifestyle and so is the consistency, if you are showing up everyday for your own self then you will definitely see yourself changing. Let's say if you eat right for one week and then just because you don't see a considerate amount of change and you give up exercising and eating right and go back to your old habits. Then all your hard work is in vain, you need to be consistent at least for 3 months and then you can see some good changes in your life. Consistency is the key to anything and remember, over doing or under doing will not help. What matters the most is doing it everyday and making it a part of your lifestyle for long.

Love & Accept Yourself

I have been on the heavier side of the scale for most of my life and I know how it feels when everyone fat shames you including your near and dear ones. One thing I learned is that if you are not comfortable in your skin then why would others let you be. Irrespective of how much everyone tries their best not everyone can be a size zero and I am talking about me too. It's okay not to be a certain size. You were not born just to fit into some clothes. It's good to be fit but chasing a particular dress size or weight is neither good nor healthy. Everyone wants to look beautiful physically but no one cares about their emotional health. So work towards a better version of yourself and rest all will fall in place.

Journey Goes On Forever

I hope through this book I have guided you all in the best way possible. Where you see me today is because of my consistency, dedication and lots of self love. I never gave up on myself, I believed in me every single day. Of course there were days when I felt like giving up, there are still days when I don't feel like exercising or getting out of bed, I indulge in junk foods, fall out of my healthy lifestyle but you know what - I don't quit. I do fall sometimes but I get up quickly.

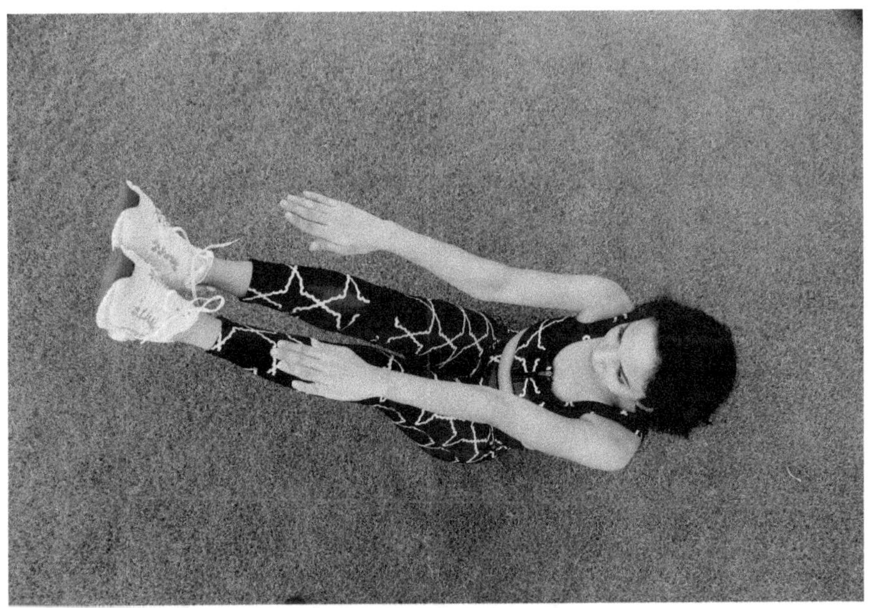

Fitness Journey Goes On

We all are human and we all tend to make mistakes. But don't let those mistakes define who you are. Now when someone asks me - what are you still trying to achieve as you are so lean and to be specific I am now 47 kgs of weight but I am not trying to lose weight anymore. I am trying to stay fit, I am trying to gain more strength, I am trying to become more flexible and there is no way I am going back. I still push myself when it's needed and I know my life purpose isn't about maintaining a certain dress size. I want to stay happy in and out and I do what makes me happy.

To all of you reading this, love yourself. From today onwards put yourself first, do what makes you happy and trust me your body will change with time. Appreciate every little thing your body can do and you will see the difference. I am like any of you, had my struggles but still managed to get that body which I always dreamt of and lastly I would say "If I Can Do It You Can Too".

In case you want any help in your fitness journey, I offer personlized services for women only:

- I am a certified nutritionist & I help my clients look better & stay healthy with my diet plans. I create all diet plans personally and will not ever give my clients valuable health to any hired staff so in case you want me to be your diet planner too, visit www.CreativeRitu.com and click on "Get Diet Plan" from menu to subscribe to your choice of diet plan. As I personally look after diets of my clients, the slots are limited.

- I understand how hard it is to motivate yourself to be physically active at home and that is why, I offer one on one personal virtual fitness training. If you would like to book visit www.CreativeRitu.com and click on "Book One On One Virtual Fitness Training" from menu to book your training. As I personally cater to my clients, the slots are limited and are mostly booked so if you are interested in working out with me personally and see a slot available (booking open on the website), book as soon as possible.

- Join me on my instagram page @mommychasingfitness & let's be fit together with regular tips & updates directly posted by me and my team.

And if there is anything else that you would like to discuss with me, feel free to email my team at support@creativeritu.com and depending upon what your query is, you will get a response (if it needs my personal response my team will let me know and I will get back to you personally as well).

I wish you all the very best in your life and fitness journey. Stay happy, fit & beautiful.

Nutritionist Ritu Dubey

Web: www.CreativeRitu.com

Email: support@creativeritu.com

Social Media: www.Instagram.com/mommychasingfitness